Relapse, Remission and Stability:

The 3 Stages Of Bipolar Disorder

Sylvia Meier

Limits of Liability / Disclaimer of Warranty:

The authors of this information and the accompanying materials have used their best efforts in preparing this course. The authors make no representation or warranties with respect to the accuracy, applicability, fitness, or completeness of the contents of this course. They disclaim any warranties (expressed or implied), merchantability, or fitness for any particular purpose. The authors shall in no event be held liable for any loss or other damages, including but not limited to special, incidental, consequential, or other damages.

DEDICATION

Relapse, remission and stability. I dedicate this book to all those people who understand all too well those terms. I dedicate this book to those of us who live within those terms.

I also dedicate this book to all those who support us during relapse, remission and stability.

The dedication also goes out to those who have loved, lost and re-found themselves in among the shambles of those stages.

This book is dedicated to everyone out there that helps others live with their bipolar worlds, and those living within them.

Sylvia Meier

CONTENTS

Introduction:

Learning to live with an illness your entire life can be hard. It takes it's toll on you and everyone you know. You learn very quickly that your life in many ways revolves around your illness.

This is very true in my life.

If I am in relapse, life is unstable, things a little crazy and I can only hope for the best.

Stability and remission go hand in hand. When you are stable, you are in remission. Your illness no longer has you by the throat on a roller coaster ride you never wanted to be on.

So many things can threaten and change where you are in the cycle.

Medications can suddenly stop working, or the side effect just become too severe to live with.

Stress can overtake you.

A single night of bad sleep can restart a cycle that ensures from that day on you get the best sleep you can.

Changing your habits or routines can do it.

Changing how you eat.

Dealing with addictions and other such issues can do it.

The list really goes on and on. Simple little things we all too often take for granted can be exactly the tipping point we needed (or wish we didn't have) to cause a change from remission to relapse, stability to instability and back and fourth on the roller coaster we go.

Then of course, relapse has to take into consideration the ups and downs of mania and depression and suddenly I hope you are getting the big picture, the picture you'll see throughout this book.

Relapse, Remission, Stability. Life with bipolar disorder.

Chapter One:

I suppose the best place to start all of this is to determine what each of those words in the title mean, I mean, what they really mean.

Webster's Dictionary defines relapse:

Suffer deterioration after a period of improvement.

Pretty simple hey? Pretty self-explanatory. Deterioration after a period of improvement. Or deterioration after a period of remission and stability. But let's not get ahead of ourselves quite yet.

Webster's Dictionary defines remission:

The cancellation of a debt, charge, or penalty

A diminution of the seriousness or intensity of disease or pain; a temporary recovery.

Again, makes sense. Pretty easy to understand. A diminution in the seriousness or intensity of disease or a temporary recovery.

So in bipolar disorder terms, things aren't quite as bad as they normally would be. Or how they are during periods of relapse. We will get much more in depth with that though.

Webster's Dictionary defines stability:

The state of being stable.

How I hate when they use the word or a derivative of the word in the definition of it. So let's take it a step back, what is stable?

Webster's Dictionary defines stable:

Not likely to change or fail; firmly established: "a stable relationship"; "prices have remained relatively stable".

So stability in terms of bipolar disorder means that you are not likely to change. You are not likely to swap from being in a state of remission back to a state of relapse.

You are stable. At least for the time being.

Chapter Two:

Relapse. Such an awful word. Reminds me of addictions. Reminds me of failure. Makes me think all sorts of unpleasant thoughts.

It's also my current state in the bipolar disorder cycle.

I am in relapse.

My stability is shot.

My medications are being played with in hopes of putting me back in remission. Back on stable ground.

It's a scary place to be. Relapse.

Just the word itself sounds scary.

Sounds like something I don't want.

And in reality, that is exactly what it is. A state of mind, and being in which I do not want to be.

It's the worse state of bipolar disorder there is.

You're up, you're down, you're spinning round and round. You can be manic, you can be hypo-manic. You can be depressed, you can be in a state of mind that feels like you are losing your mind.

It's a very hard place to be.

So what happens when you are in this state.

Well, a whole lot.

Like I already mentioned your moods can be all over the place.

For me right now it is manifesting itself in a whole lot of swings. Like an insane amount of mood swings. I can be amazingly happy and content, and in the very next moment I am crying my eyes out. Like bawling my eyes out. Only to seconds later be laughing at something that really shouldn't be that funny, but for some reason, some strange reason, it is the funniest thing I have heard in my life, till my cheeks hurt from laughing. And I start to cry again.

Back and fourth it goes.

This is my relapse.

I hold hope though, for the time being (there will be-oots later I am sure that feel hopeless, like I will never regain stability ever again) that I will re-stabilize, that my disorder, my illness, the creature that controls much of my life will descend back into remission so that maybe, just maybe I can go back to a stable happy place again.

Entry One:

Today is one of those days I wonder how I function sometimes at all.

Everything is taking so much effort today.

Just the kitchen floor was enough to drive me crazy and send me to tears. Not sure what the kids spilled all over it, all I know is no matter what I do or try it won't stop feeling gross. Not sure if it's just me, cause no one else seems to notice.

Watching a little man graduate kindergarten was bittersweet. He's the last of the bunch. I'll never see another kindergarten graduation, I'll never have another pre-

schooler and even though I swore today I wouldn't cry, I was in tears hugging the founder of the special needs school little man went to... went to.

I've been writing most of the day. Only place I can seem to catch my focus, and even that is coming with some effort.

See the psychiatrist and psychologist in the morning.

Perhaps they can help me down off the roller-coaster. Cause I don't wanna be on it anymore. Never wanted to be on it to begin with. Stupid medication, had to make me puke, had to stop working.

I hate medications. Wish they worked forever. Wished this illness went into remission FOREVER and that I was stable forever, or at least for the most part.

I'm starting to develop a very much love hate relationship with this illness. On one hand it gives me mania and hypo-mania which at times are just peachy and make it so I can get unbelievable amounts of things done.

Other times I hate it. Like today. I hate it. I don't wanna be unable to function.

Why can't I function today? So cannot function and it's pissing me off.

I had so much planned to do today and instead I have stared at blank screens, refreshed pages that will never change and scrubbed the floor 3 different times. Plus watched a little man graduate and lost myself to tears. Uggh.

This is relapse. This is instability. This is the part of being bipolar and having this damn disorder that sucks. That pisses me off. That makes me hate it. Grrr.

That is relapse. This is relapse. I am in the heart of a relapse. I was in remission for give or take 8 months. Been battling with medications for the last 3-4 months now.

I really do hate the word relapse though. It's a tainted word. It feels dirty to me. I didn't choose this.

Yes, some people choose relapse. Some people with the disorder are so out of sorts when the ups and downs stop, or when the mania never comes back that they self sabotage the healing process and do things like stopping medications and therapies. They would rather have the ups and downs of a relapse, of an episode then the stability that comes with remission.

It's a hard battle that's for sure. Finding an even ground where you are okay with who you are and how you feel, while maintaining stability.

There's no real way to describe it to someone who hasn't lived it. On one hand you want to relapse and return to things like being manic and the energy and good stuff that comes with mania and on the other hand you never want to see that side of yourself again. At least that's how I feel. Yes, I love my Miss Manic, but a large part of me hates her with all my heart and soul. I look back at the things I've done as her, or she's done and cringe. I shake my head and want to cry, which is usually what happens because by the time Miss Manic leaves my Quiet Girl, my depression has hit full force.

That again is relapse. Traveling back and forth between the two stages, with very little time on level ground.

Uggh. This is relapse.

This is what people need to understand from the point of someone living with it. It's hard, it makes us grouchy and unreliable, it sends our moods all over the place and we know it is hard on those that love us and care for us, but it is just as hard on us and we don't know how to stop it, or make it better. Only thing we can do is hope someone on our medical team can come up with a solution to rope us back to stable ground, to send this evil little illness back into remission so we can continue on with our lives stable.

Entry Two:

Today is a little better. I feel like I can again take on the world. Though things may seem a little bit crazy, a little more hectic than I would really care for I don't feel hopeless. I feel like I can actually handle this illness again.

Maybe it's optimism in the face of adversity.

Maybe it's knowing in a few hours I see two of the members of my medical team and perhaps they'll have some ideas to pull this roller-coaster to a halt. Who knows how I'll feel if they are as clueless as I am right now as to what to do.

The rain though is killing me. I know my mood and everything wants to come back up but the downpour outside is fighting my mood, making me feel tired and worn out. Or maybe I simply am tired and worn out.

Haven't really slept well in nights. Last night was better but it was still awful. I simply wish sometimes I could sleep like a normal person (gawd I hate that term, what the hell is normal exactly, cause this is normal for me and most of the bipolar population) and go to bed, know that I will be able to sleep and wake up in the morning functioning.

Instead I go to bed, not knowing whether or not I will get a wink of sleep or I will sleep so deep as not to wake even with the alarm clock ringing through my head. Then of course it comes down to the morning mood. Most of the time I can tell how the day will go. Today I'm not sure. I was great waking up, cuddling with my girlfriend before escaping the covers, seeing her off to work, then it all falls apart.

The rain sucks. It's too much. My shoes are leaking water and my feet are soaked before I even hit the car. The steering wheel is fighting me when I try to turn. I trip UP the stairs leaving my little man's classroom, and on I am sure the day will go.

This is just another day of relapse, this is just another day of hoping for remission.

And relapse simply continues in that fashion. The ups and downs, the back and fourth, the mind altering roller-coaster that makes you wonder when you will ever put your feet back on solid ground. When will you ever be stable again?

Entry Three:

The lack of sleep seems to be getting to me. It's making my mopey and lackluster. The weather sure is playing it's role too. It's hard to look out at the rain and gloomy weather and not feel blah. And of course the fact we have record breaking flooding and the whole world seems to be upside down doesn't help in any manner. Ah, so is the life though.

I'm still struggling with my moods. I feel like I will always struggle. I would simply like to get back some stability, some little form of solid ground.

Even my writing is suffering. I was doing really well. I was writing at a normal pace, I was completing things that needed to be completed. I was living life. Then the stupid medication decided not to want to co-operate. Not to allow my stomach to keep it down. The smell alone was killer, couldn't handle even the smell. And back on the roller coaster I went. It wasn't so bad at the start. I was slightly hypo-manic. I was getting more stuff done. I was getting things around the house going. I was living, albeit in a little faster pace then I should have been. Hell, I even wrote almost 6 books. I say almost 6 books, cause this is the sixth one. I got caught on another one and it swept away my wind for writing. It threw it out the window. To tough a topic to write about yet I think, too fuzzy a topic perhaps. So I moved on. And I write this book. This entry. And wonder what tomorrow will bring.

I hope and pray for stability again. I loved it. It was a peaceful state of mind. It was a good place to be. It was... good.

I'll just keep going with what the doctors say and hope one of these days the hit and miss game of medication is a hit again and I can resume my life, without the roller-coaster.

Sylvia Meier

Chapter 3:

Remission.

As I already stated previously, I hate this word.

Bipolar disorder is not cancer. I don't think it is something that goes into remission. You will always have it. Remission is just an unpleasant word to me to describe stability. I would much rather have them use the word stability as a state of the disorder then remission.

Anyways, onto remission we go.

Remission is that thing you long for when you are deep in the depths of depression. It's the time you wish for as you're propelling off the ledge of the inevitable crash. It's not something you ever want when caught in mania's throes.

Mania is a mistress who holds you tight, whispers your own invincibility in your ears, makes your ego swoon and sends you off on the trip of your life, globe-trotting, running half-naked through the streets, high on life, most likely drugs and anything else you've shoved into your body since it began.

The last thing a manic person is thinking about is remission. Hell, they probably aren't even thinking about relapse because by the time you are there you are so far gone, you've forgotten about sanity, because you, your Miss Manic is the epitome of everything you've ever wanted in your life and more. Stability is the last thing on her mind because she believes herself stable and at the top of her game. She is queen (or he is king) of the universe and nothing anyone else has to say will change that.

Mania was always something I loved when in relapses where I went manic but was never a time where I found myself wishing for stability. I thought myself stable. I thought everything in my world alright and it was the furthest thing from the truth.

I've had the odd period of remission and it is often like awakening from a nightmare. Whether coming into it from mania or depression it feels like you've awakened from a coma and are seeing everything that happened in your life while you were away. Except unlike being in a coma, you were there for it all. You may not have seen it as destruction and chaos as it occurred, but once in remission your eyes are opened and you realize just how far up or down you had gotten.

For me the first major remission of my life took place after coming off the psych ward. This is true of most others. It takes things getting that bad for you to be finally able to stop, sort yourself out in the ward and come back to life hopefully with some degree of stability.

I will admit when I first walked out the doors of the psych ward I was anything but stable. I was no longer a threat to myself but stable was not me. I was still an utter mess. It took a couple weeks of soul searching, a ton of support and a lot of reading for me to start feeling stable. It took probably a month or two back in the real world before stability started to set in and even then there were set-backs. Just like anyone without the disorder, there are good and bad days. There are days where you know you're in remission, that you're stable and going to be able to stay there and there are other days you doubt your new found feet and fall to the ground like a child taking her first steps.

And much like that child taking their first steps, that is what stability and remission is. It is a step at a time, a day at a time, a moment at a time, and each one builds on the one prior until before you know it you're on your feet running and stable as can be.

That is, till you fall back down again. Till you lose your

footing. And no one knows how badly bruised and scraped up you'll be with that fall. For sometimes you'll be able to dust yourself off and get back in the race, and other times you fall so hard, relapse swallows you whole and your out of the race again and back on the roller-coaster.

This is bipolar disorder. This is relapse, this is remission, this is stability, this is my bipolar world.

I'd love nothing else then to place an entry here showing what I am like during a stable period but because stability is so few and far between and as I write this book I am in the heart of a relapse instead I will try my best to describe who I am, how I feel and where my mind is at when I am stable.

When stable I can handle things that occur in life without it being too simple. I mean, when manic, I can take on the world, nothing it throws my way could ever be too difficult for me to handle. Nothing that comes into my life, or needs to be handled is too hard to handle.

Hand it to me in a depression and it will swallow me whole. Even the simplest of problems are overwhelming. Simple things like trying to get out of bed are difficult. Like really difficult.

Stability then is being able to handle the things that occur in life, without being over confident in my abilities, and that things will work out just fine.

Stability also means a normal sleep pattern.

Depression means I want to do nothing more than sleep day in and day out. Mania means I don't need sleep, like any sleep, ever. Even when I have been awake for 7 straight days and not had hardly a wink.

Stability means I eat regular healthy meals.

Depression means I eat far too much, and of all the wrong stuff. With mania I have no appetite or am famished all the time, but again it's anything but the food I should be putting into my body (and boy does my body rebel about it.)

Stability means, that well, I'm stable.

Both in depression and mania my moods are all over the place. They really are up and down in both ends of their spectrum and they leave me feeling like I am losing my mind (which is very much a reality when in depression and mania, I've already lost my mind, I just don't know it yet.)

It means that I have control over my emotions to a relative degree. I'm not crying cause I cannot get the floor to clean. I am not stupid happy, and in tears of laughter over nothing at all. I am not staying up day and night thinking the world is a okay and I will be able to do everything I ever dreamed up. My emotions match the situation instead of residing in an all or nothing state of mind.

Stability, really, means a lot. It means the whole world to someone who is bipolar and aware of their illness. It means everything to someone who has been there, has lost it and knows they have lost it. It means everything to someone who was happy living stable. It means the world to someone who lives in a bipolar world, but no longer wants to ride the roller-coaster.

Stability means remission and remission means stability, and both would be the greatest thing in the world for me to feel again. You see as I write this, I'm anything but stable. As I write this I am deep in the battle of relapse, but aware enough that I really would like to go back to living outside that realm, where I am stable and live makes sense, my emotions make sense, all of it makes sense again as it once did.

Stability really does mean the world to someone who has lost it. It means the world to someone like me who would really like to see life through stable eyes again. Who would like to be able to look at the world with stable mind and understand and look at things the way they are supposed to be.

As much as I hate the word, stable would also mean feeling like I was normal again. I will never really be normal in the typical sense of the word because I am someone who is quite unique, but it would be as close to normal as I would want to get. It would mean normal with a slight twist and a cocktail of pills.

Stable would mean happiness to me. It would mean being able to wake up and knowing how I would feel that day. It would mean not being afraid to do my make-up because there is no point if everything would simply bring me to tears for no reason again. It would mean knowing that when I awoke I could make plans for the day and not be afraid that things would go awry like it seems to do so much these days.

Stable, in conclusion would mean so very much.

Sylvia Meier

Conclusion:

Conclusions are getting tough. It never feels like there should be a conclusion because I know there is another book, or two, or five within me.

That said, I hope this book has given you another look into my bipolar world. I hope it enlightens you and makes you understand the illness just a little more, whether you are the one who has it, or are someone who has a loved one with it.

I hope you learn that even though there are all these industry terms and definitions, what is something for one person will or will not be the same for the very next person.

I hope you walk away with more knowledge within your mind and heart of what it truly is to live with bipolar disorder. What it is really like to live with such a life-altering disorder that can take your life in a moment, or send you to the moon with mania in another.

I've come to hate endings, and the conclusions, so instead I bid farewell, and promise you my return with another book, still directed to the walk of my life, and my bipolar world and hope that you wonderful reader, will join me in that book as well.

Sylvia Meier

Other Books By Sylvia Meier

Living Bipolar: Learning To Live With Bipolar Disorder

http://www.amazon.com/Living-Bipolar-My-World-ebook/dp/B00CP58BLI/

http://www.amazon.com/Living-Bipolar-Learning-Live-Disorder/dp/1484816366/

Bipolar Bits: Manic Madness To Depressive Depths

http://www.amazon.com/Bipolar-Bits-Madness-Depressive-ebook/dp/B00CW667IY/

http://www.amazon.com/Bipolar-Bits-Madness-Depressive-Depths/dp/1484990722/

Lotta Bipolar Bits: Survivors Diary Of Living Bipolar

http://www.amazon.com/Lotta-Bipolar-Bits-Survivors-ebook/dp/B00D2VZ3TW/

http://www.amazon.com/Lotta-Bipolar-Bits-Survivors-Living/dp/1489589368/

My Bipolar World: A Collection Of Works By Sylvia Meier

http://www.amazon.com/My-Bipolar-World-Collection-ebook/dp/B00D2XY8QO/

http://www.amazon.com/My-Bipolar-World-Collection-Sylvia/dp/1489517030

Bipolar Hope: Discovering Hope In Your Diagnosis

http://www.amazon.com/Bipolar-Hope-Discovering-Diagnosis-ebook/dp/B00D9WSLUC

http://www.amazon.com/Bipolar-Hope-Discovering-Diagnosis-World/dp/1490370706

Relapse, Remission and Stability: The 3 Stages Of Bipolar Disorder

COMING SOON:

- **The Psych Ward: Losing To Bipolar Disorder And Starting Life Again**

- **My Bipolar World: A Second Collection Of Works By Sylvia Meier**

- **Support And Bipolar: You Need More Than Just You**

- **The Claws And Embrace: Depression In Bipolar Disorder**

- **Manic, Misery And More: The Upswing Of Living Bipolar**

- **My Bipolar World: A Third Collection Of Works By Sylvia Meier**

ABOUT THE AUTHOR

I'm not doing this about the author is traditional fashion. It's awkward and plain strange to write about myself in the third person.

My name is Sylvia.

I'll be 32 this summer.

I am the mother of 5 beautiful children.

I am the partner of the beautiful woman who has been my greatest support in my fight.

I am living bipolar. I have bipolar disorder type one. I was first diagnosed at 13 years old, and went through the typical denial and rebellion.

Fast forward 17 years and life is off-kilter, all sorts of wrong, my illness has left my life shattered, tattered and my life on a string.

Suicide attempt, stopped by myself was the best and worst moment of my life. It was the wake up call I needed, and the scare I needed. I took my illness in my hands, decided to be in control instead of my disorder being in control and here I am a year later in the best mental health of my life.

I won't lie, there are days that are tough, there are days I long to be manic again. Overall though, I am happy, I am healthy and I have more support in my life than I could ever imagine.

I am a writer by passion. This is not my first book and surely will not be my last. I am in the process of writing another one called "Woman Broken, A Child Lost" which is about my life, my struggles and everything in between. It too will hopefully be out this year, but is one of those stories that will not be released until perfection is reached as it is my story. My full story.

I do also have another book out called "Living Bipolar" which you can find in kindle version and print on my site at http://www.MyBipolarWorld.com/livingbipolar.html .

Till then you can always find me and support for yourself on my website which is my story and writings as well. Check it out at http://www.MyBipolarWorld.com

In the end, I send you all much love and hope. If you take nothing else from all of this at least know you are not alone, and if you ever need that ear, feel free to contact me at my site. I do my best to respond to everyone as time and living bipolar allows.

Love,
  Sylvia

www.ingramcontent.com/pod-product-compliance
Lightning Source LLC
Chambersburg PA
CBHW070528290526
45790CB00003B/1344